Thank you God for giving me the grit and grind
in the midst of grief to get it done.

For I know the plans I have for you Kim, declares
the Lord, plans to prosper you and not to harm
you, plans to give you a hope and a future.

JEREMIAH 29 V 11 NIV

LET'S GET IT DONE!

Copyright 2017 by Kimberly Griffin

Editing: ZION Publishing House

Creative Director: Katie Brady Design

ISBN: 978-1543171754

Printed In The United States of America.

Dedication

Often times when you pick up a book it is dedicated to someone else and not you. Guess what? This one is for you! Just because we haven't met doesn't mean I don't know who you are. We are the same because we have had the same struggles and fought the same fights in life in one area or another. We may never meet, but you are always on my mind. So here's to you! Let's run to the finish line. WE GOT THIS!

A Fuel Your Tank Moment With Kim

There were times I would be in the gym parking lot, wanting to put the car in reverse and go back home. But God would encourage me and tell me things He knew my heart needed to hear at that moment. Those words gave me the strength to move past what I was feeling and helped me remember what I was committed to. My journey was never for me; it was always for those whom I was destined to serve. Every time I would reach a victory in the gym, someone's life would be changed. I realized that my health and fitness journey became someone else's fuel to stop them from giving up or "throwing in the towel." During my journey, I began to realize that people who I didn't know were watching me and were getting inspired to begin their own journeys. Those same people gave me the fire I needed to go above and beyond what I sought out to do each day. I believe in you, and I pray that these thirty days will change your life and cause a ripple effect to those who you encounter, starting in your own home. Park your excuses and get ready for a premium fill up, and Let's Get It Done!

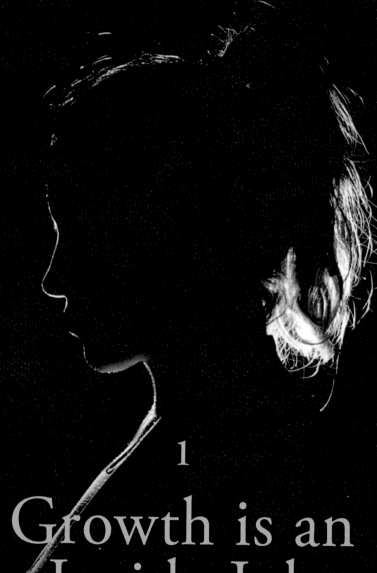

1
Growth is an Inside Job

First, let's deal with any mental hindrances that will cause you not to go for it! Growth is truly an inside job. Once you make the change on the inside, you will be able to see success on the outside. Travel on the inside before you can travel on the outside.

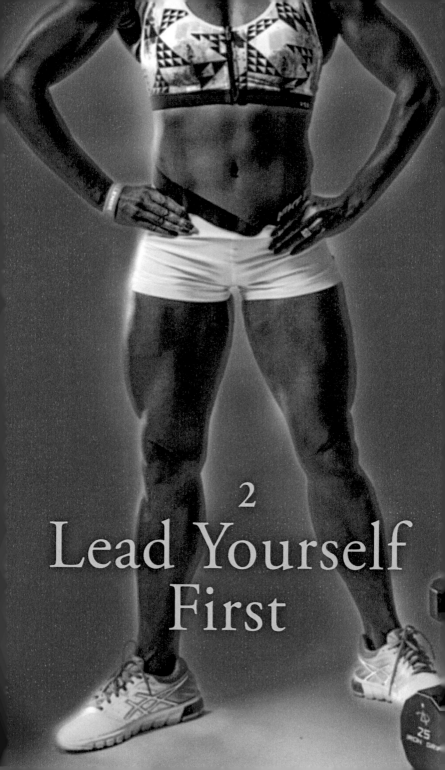

2
Lead Yourself
First

The first person you lead in your journey is yourself. An important attribute to work on that's common to all great leaders is self-discipline. Once you master self-discipline, you will be able to lead others in your journey.

3
Make Discipline a Lifestyle

Make a disciplined lifestyle your goal. Change is not a one time event nor can it be emotionally based. Consider developing a routine and follow it daily. Remember, there is no such thing as failure while you are attempting to establish a routine. Struggles will simply expose areas you need more discipline in. A disciplined lifestyle is to be desired.

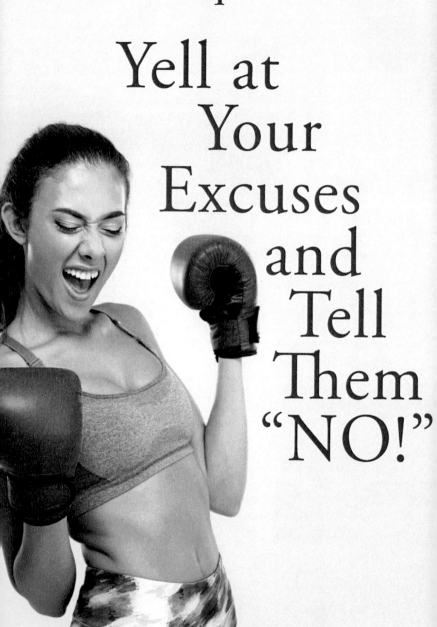

4

Yell at Your Excuses and Tell Them "NO!"

Challenge your excuses
and pay attention to your
tendencies. If you are full of
excuses, YOU are the barrier
to your success and no one
else. If you want to go to the
next level, challenge yourself
and yell at your excuses.
NOW YELL:
"YOU CAN'T STOP ME!"

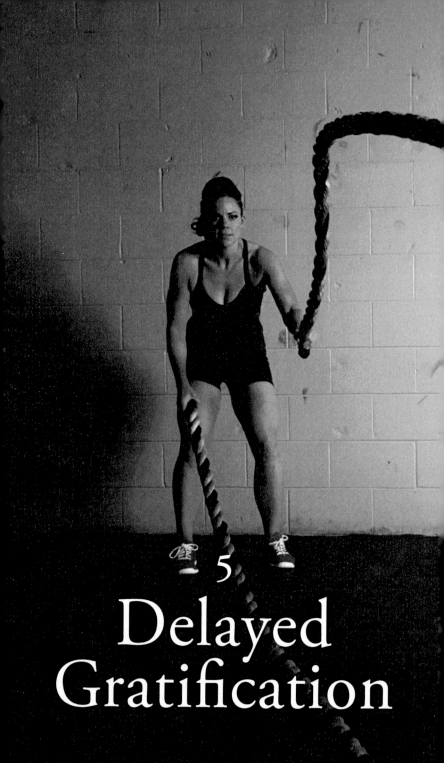

5
Delayed
Gratification

Remove the rewards until you finish the job. Consider celebrating at the end not during the process. You can't afford to have a huge celebration without a huge victory. Losing twelve pounds does not equal celebrating with twelve cookies!
Keep pushing, "Champ."
If you want to celebrate a milestone along the way during your journey, go and buy yourself the next size smaller in clothing.

6

Can You See Yourself Smaller?

Stop looking at the size you are in the mirror and imagine yourself smaller. Perhaps, get an old picture of yourself and see yourself smaller. Lock that vision into your mind, and see yourself as that until it manifests. You are not who you currently see in the mirror; instead you are who you envision and believe you will become.

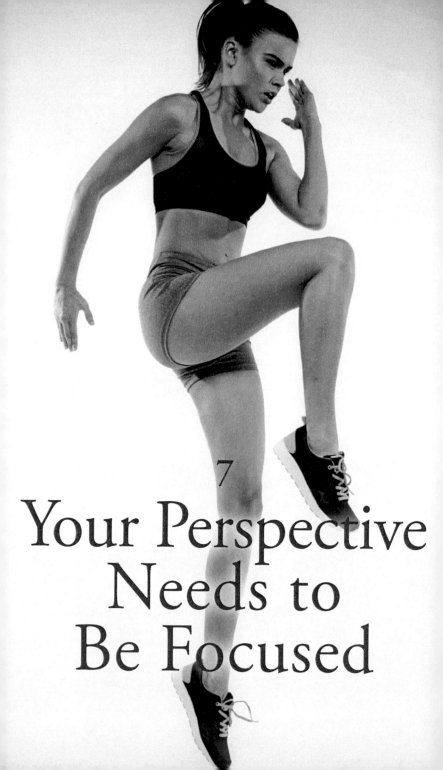

7

Your Perspective Needs to Be Focused

Shift your focus! Stay focused on results instead of focusing on what you are giving up. Think of what you are gaining, so you don't become discouraged during the process. Change your perspective and dive in with your mind set on victory. Believe and go for it!

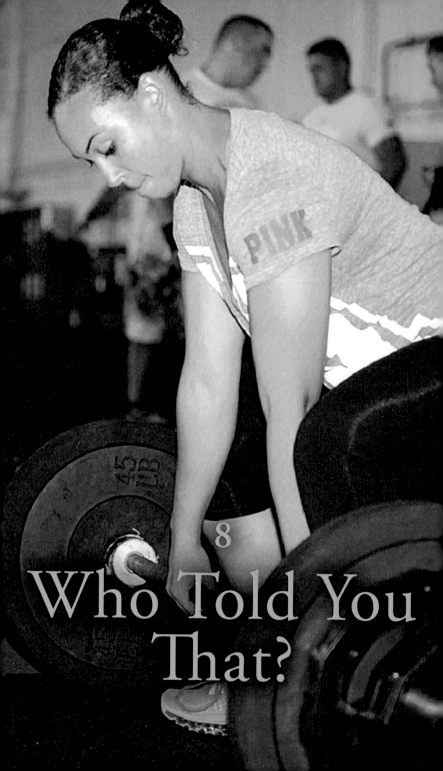

8

Who Told You That?

Who told you that you couldn't do it? Who told you it would take over a year? Where is the negativity coming from? Guess what? As you begin to gain healthy habits, your circle will change. Your new friends will begin to tell you great and encouraging things to help you cross the finish line. Silence any negativity and get busy.

9
You Are Your Best Friend

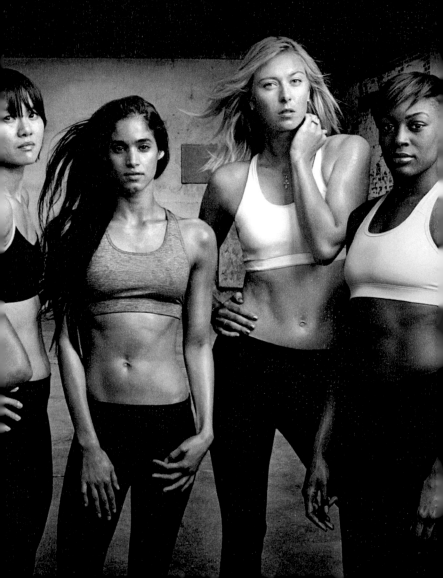

No need to have a gym partner with you all the time. At some point, your schedules won't work, or you will be working on two different body parts at the gym. Instead, get a "Fit Squad." This squad will simply give you a high five and offer great words of encouragement. At some point, you should graduate to encouraging yourself on your personal journey. Remember, who you started with may not be who you finish with. You have what it takes; now let's go get it!

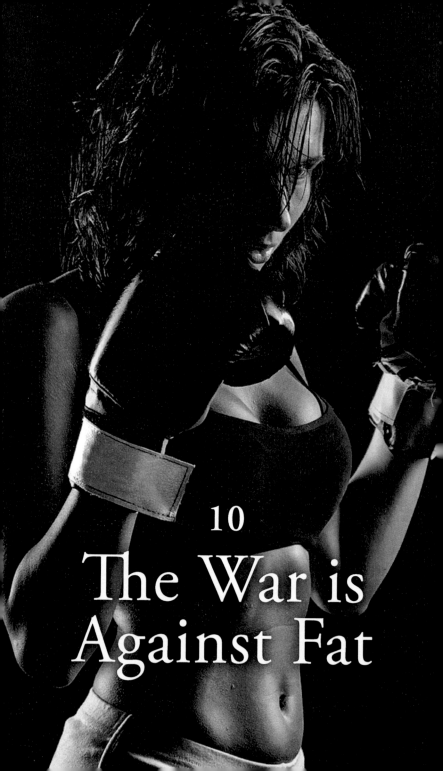

10

The War is Against Fat

Fat is sneaky and easy to get on but hard to get off. When you start your workout, set your mind for battle. You are battling to win against that body fat. Put the pedal to the medal and fight. It's a war going on and guess what? **YOU WIN!**

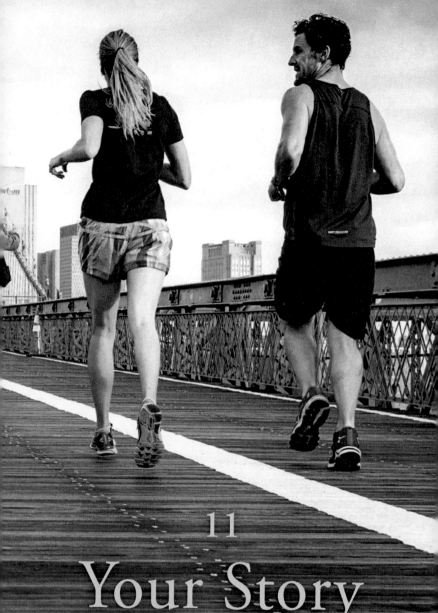

11

Your Story
Matters

People are watching you because you are showing up everyday and are looking different. Be mindful to speak to people and start a friendly conversation. To be honest with you, they'll be glad you did because you will have given them hope. They need to hear your story! Share your true and authentic story. It will bring hope and change a life. Remember, you were once in their shoes.

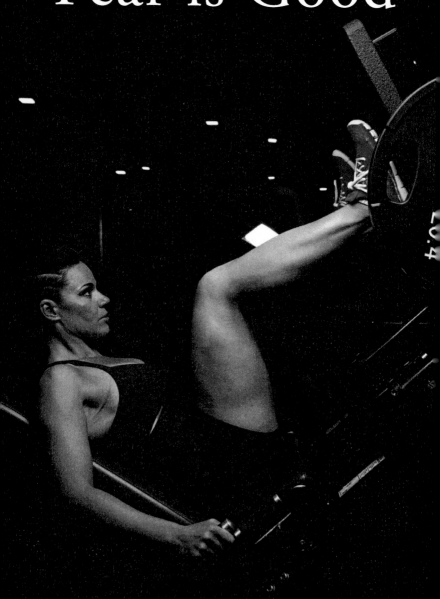

12
Fear is Good

To not live in fear is not living at all. Fear of the unknown is good. Along your journey of transformation, you will find yourself and discover that what you once feared does not exist and is not true.

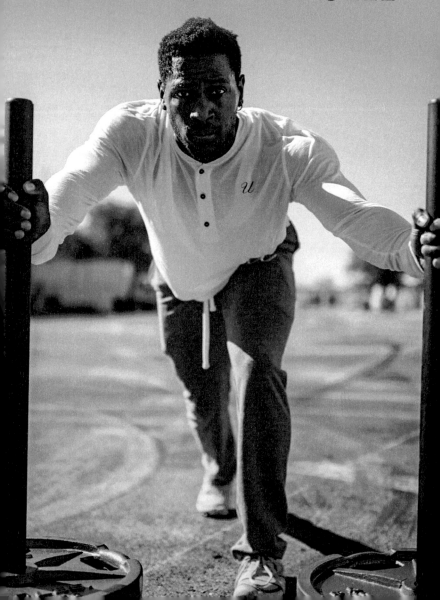

13
Who Cares About Them

What people think about you is none of your business; it has nothing to do with you. While your haters are doing what they do, you continue to conquer your goals, follow your passion, serve people, and be free! Smile and laugh. You can't be stopped!

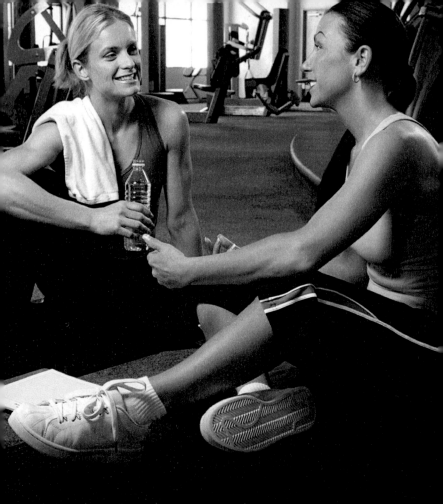

14
Encourage
Somebody

The next time you see someone having a hard time on the treadmill, just give them a "high five" and say, "I saw you doing an awesome job; you've got what it takes." While you are encouraging others, you'll also be encouraging yourself.

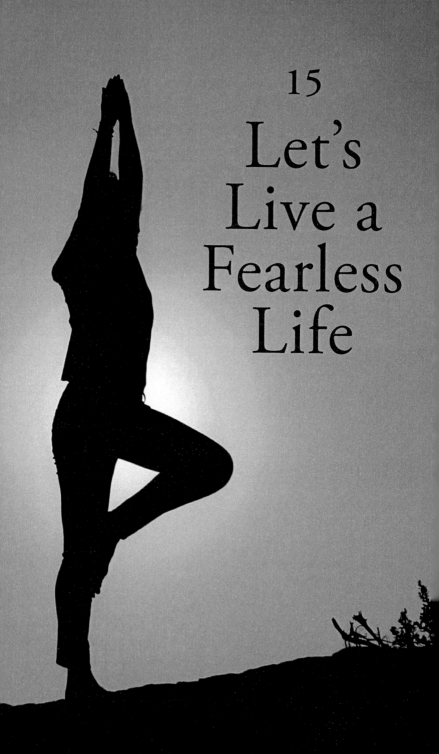

15

Let's Live a Fearless Life

Spread your wings and fly. Often times we are held in bondage of peoples' opinions of what we are doing. Break free of that and have an "I don't care what they think" kind of attitude. You will soon realize that they admired you the entire time while you are enjoying the breeze of flying in freedom.

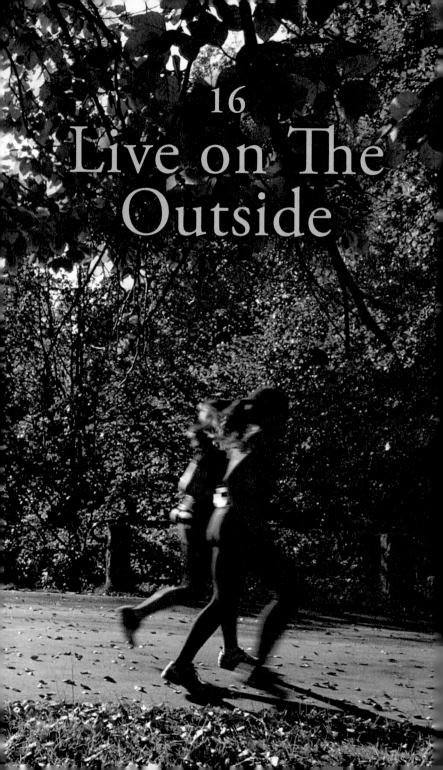

16
Live on The
Outside

Live on the outside of your comfort zone, and let's see what can be accomplished. Say to yourself, "I'm here to be uncomfortable and do something I have never done." "Now is not the time to let my heart rate relax; let's turn it up!"

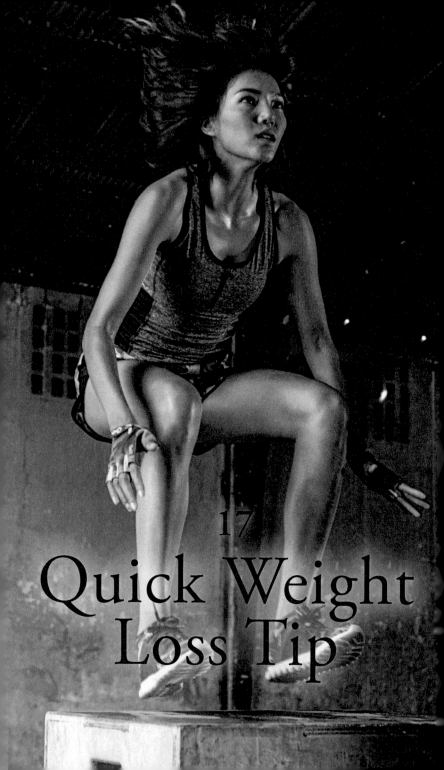

17
Quick Weight Loss Tip

You want to lose some
weight today?
Go back and apologize to
the person you are mad at,
whether you are right or wrong.
Whether they receive it or not,
truly forgive them and put the
situation in the "cemetery."
The cemetery is the place for
dead things that should not be
resurrected in thought
(i.e. playing it back in your
mind) or conversation. Take
back YOUR moments, words,
and time. Holding on to past
hurts and pain, day in and
day out, is a weight.

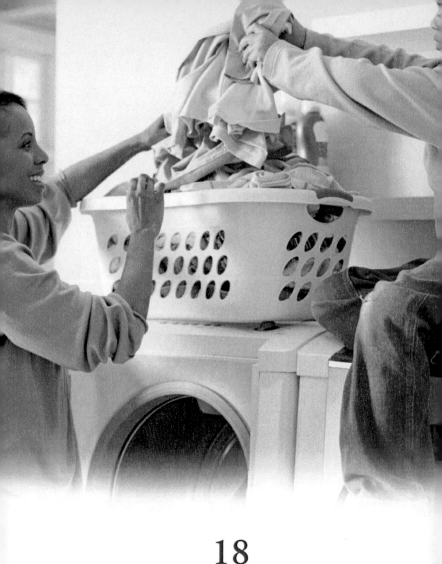

18
The Family Will be Fine

Your support system works and everyone will be fine. Make sure the homework is done, a load is in the laundry, lunches are made, dinner is given, snack are in place, and the house is in average order. Your support systems works. Now lets not try to be so much in control and so perfect at home that you neglect yourself. Trust me, once you reach your goals there will be a new you in town.

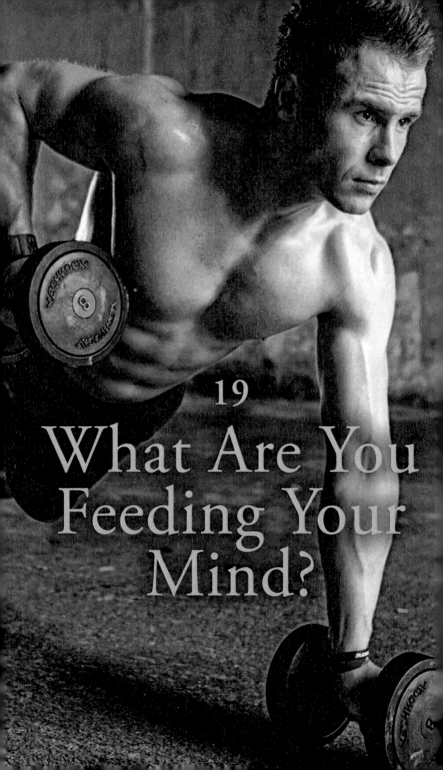

19

What Are You Feeding Your Mind?

I tell myself while working
out the following:

"3 pounds - I'm coming for you today."

"Muscles, I command you to
grow and show."

"Flesh, I control you; you don't
control me."

"I'm here now, and I am not leaving
the same way I came in; something
must go and grow."

"It's a great day to lose some fat!"

"Don't stop until you are done."

"It's me against the best Kim.
Let's fight!"

"I'm losing something today; yes I am."

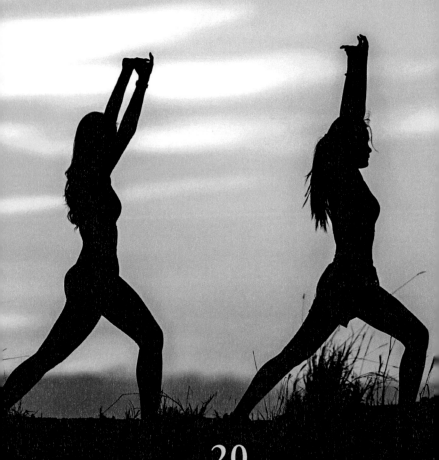

20
Consistency
Compounds

What you do day in
and day out will catch up
with you. That's awesome
news! Consistency is key,
and you must ride it like a
horse and refuse to
get off. Just like interest for
a bank account adds up,
so does your effort.

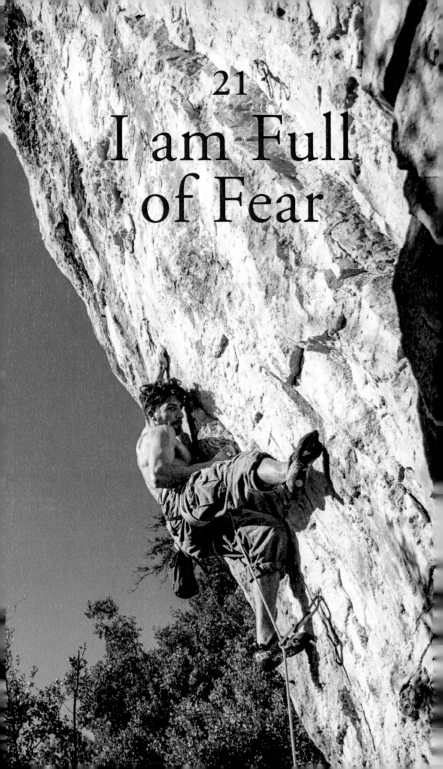

21
I am Full of Fear

Living life in fear of what you will become should be the new normal. Here is the good news! Right behind fear is your breakthrough! You are right on track to be blessed.

I'm a jumper. The cliff of the unknown won't stop me. I refuse to leave earth without discovering all of my gifts, talents, purposes, -we have more than one- and blessings. Utilize all the talents you have been given. They're for others. When people talk about you in life, will they say you are a jumper (full of faith) or a watcher (always talking about what you are about to do but never taking action)?

Speed up your journey and jump!
Tick tock.
The clock is ticking.

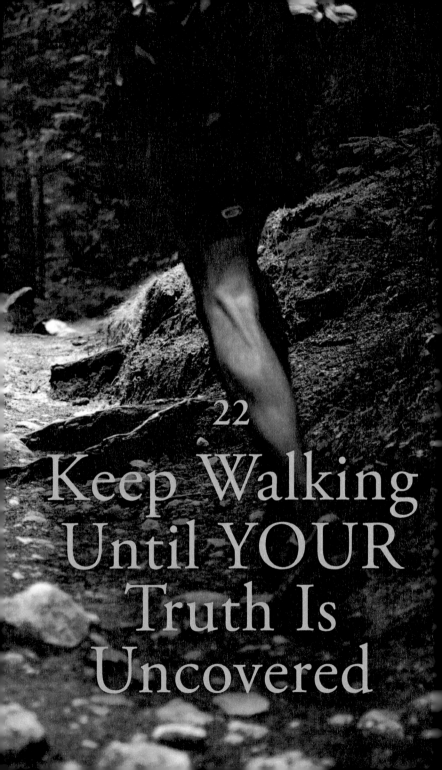

22
Keep Walking Until YOUR Truth Is Uncovered

Your truths will be discovered and uncovered as you are walking this journey out. You will begin to see that you are mentally stronger than you thought, and you have what it takes. There are some truths about you that you will discover, but they're at the finish line. Keep walking.

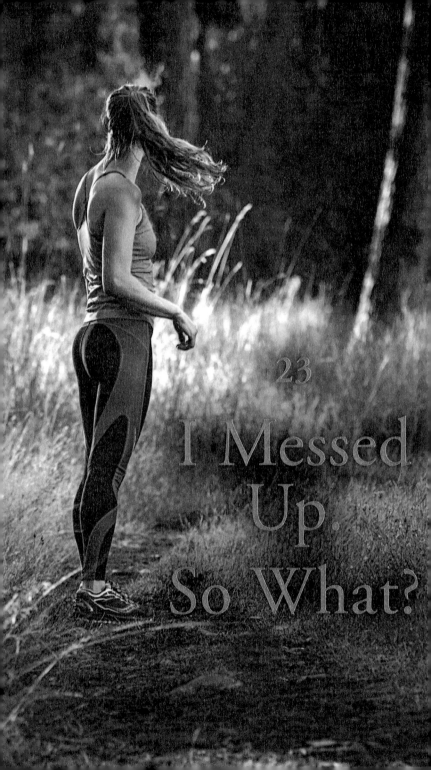

23

I Messed Up.
So What?

Who cares if you messed up?
Let's get up and keep growing
and going. Consistency
compounds but nothing can
add up if you keep stopping.
Results are waiting for you in
the morning.

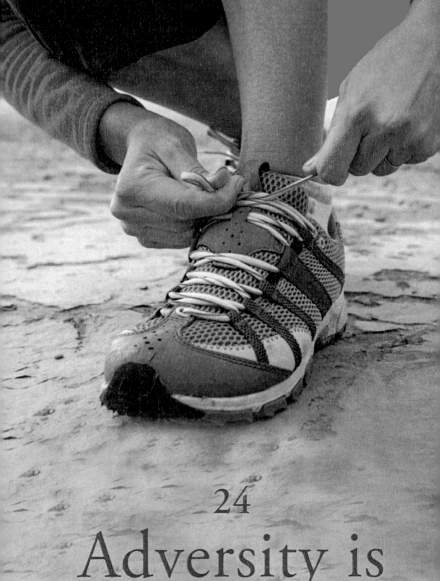

24
Adversity is Fuel

Life may happen in the midst of your journey. But it's ok. Pack up your issues and take them to the gym. Work "it" out there. If you can come through this, you are truly an elite champion. Keep climbing. You are still on a journey, and issues you may encounter are called "life." You can do it. Now, take the next step.

25
Encourage Your Competition

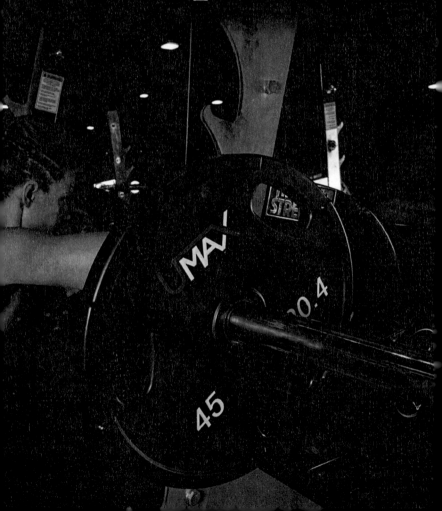

Look in the mirror. That's your competition. It's YOU! It isn't anyone else. Only you know what you have on the inside of you. Go harder, push faster, and find your wall.

R.I.P.

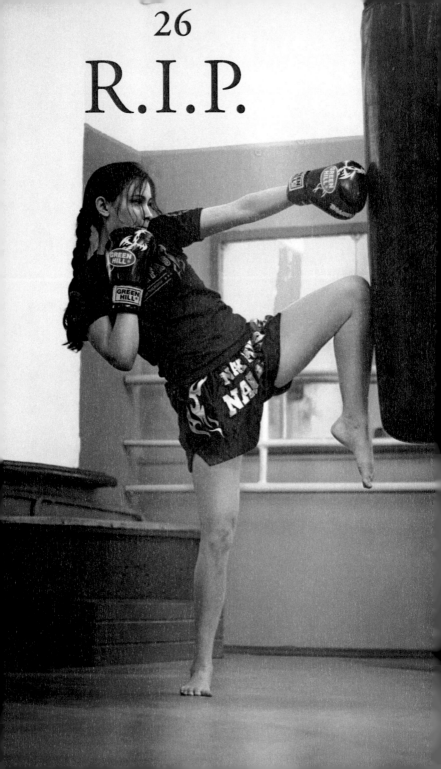

Tell your fat to Rest In Peace! There is a battle going on, and it's against fat. You must change your mindset, walking through the gym doors. Say, "Fat, be prepared to die today. I am coming after you!"

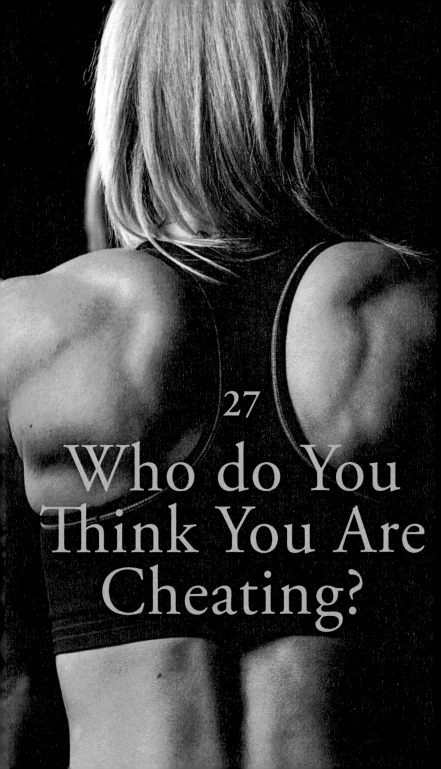

27

Who do You Think You Are Cheating?

I've got news for you!
If you didn't finish that rep,
you are cheating yourself. If
you did not finish your cardio,
you are cheating yourself.
Why are you cheating
yourself? You, alone, will
suffer the consequences and
no one else. Now, let's get
back on it and finish or
finish up in the morning.
Don't be a cheater.

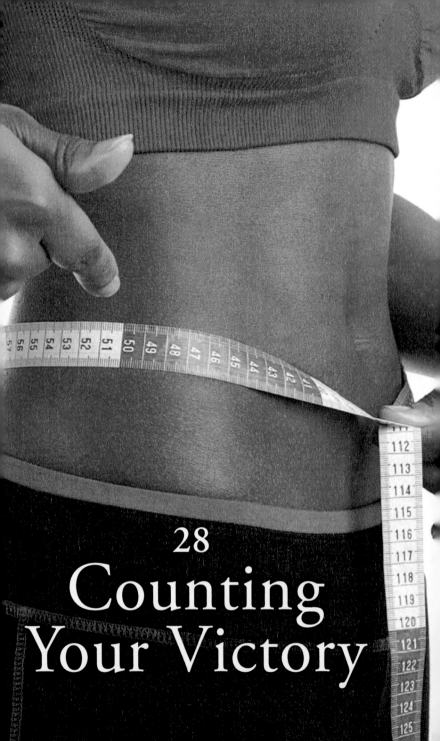

28
Counting
Your Victory

All victories do not look the same. Some will show in clothing and others will show on the scale, in addition to your attitude or perhaps your confidence. A win is a win! Keep going and keep winning because the victories get better.

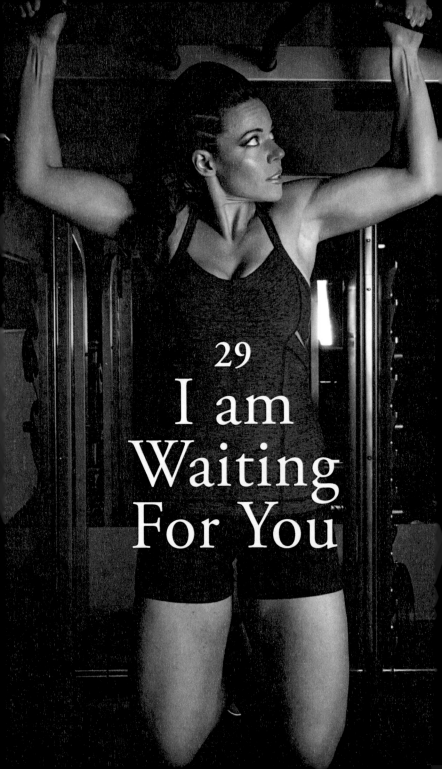

29

I am
Waiting
For You

Sit your butt back down and finish that set! Or, try and lift it and get one or two reps out. I know it's heavy, and your mind is telling you, "No," but at some point, you should push your limits. With that being said, sit down and do it. The weights have all day to wait for you.

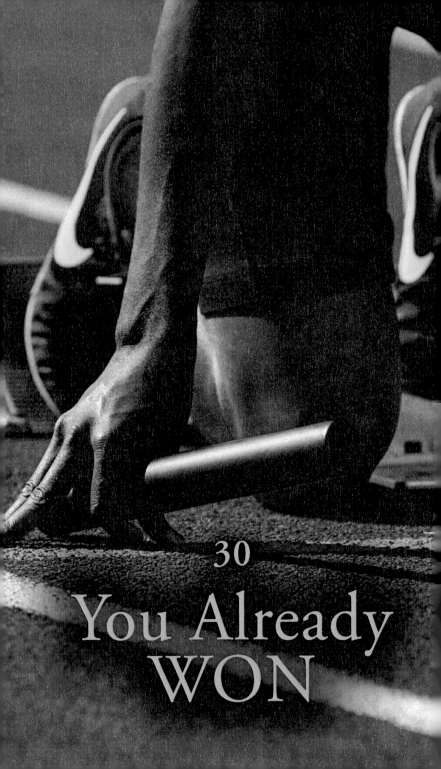

30
You Already
WON

The day you decided to start is the day you won. The average person is still trying to start something and cannot seem to take action, but you did. Congrats! You won the first step. Keep going to see your rewards. Let me be the first person to tell you this, "You are a winner!"

Please list the excuses that have stopped you currently and in the past from getting it done.

_____

_____

_____

_____

_____

_____

_____

_____

_____

_____

_____

_____

_____

_____

Positive Affirmation:
Today I acknowledge that I will be presented with numerous excuses that I can use to hold me back. I have decided not to give into the excuses and win.

Please list yours goals and add a date that you wish to accomplish them by.

_____

_____

_____

_____

_____

_____

_____

_____

_____

_____

_____

_____

_____

_____

If you have enjoyed
the motivation from this book,
Kim would love to hear from you.
Please visit her website at:
KimGriffinSpeaks.com
to post a comment

Made in the USA
San Bernardino, CA
26 February 2017